When Alzheimer's Disease Strikes!

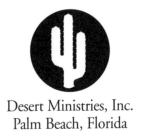

By

DR. STEPHEN SAPP

Desert Ministries, Inc.
Palm Beach, Florida

WHEN ALZHEIMER'S DISEASE STRIKES

Fifth Edition
First Printing Revised Edition, II
©Copyright 2002 by
Desert Ministries, Inc.
P.O. Box 788
Palm Beach, FL 33480
ISBN 0-914733-30-3

Printed by Eagle Graphic Services, Fort Lauderdale, Florida

✺ PUBLISHER'S PREFACE ✺

As President of Desert Ministries Inc., I am especially proud and pleased to write this little introduction to Dr. Sapp's revised and updated volume *"When Alzheimer's Disease Strikes."* Not only is Stephen a noted authority on the subject, he is a trusted friend and fellow traveler. We at DMI are grateful for his willingness to share this book through us. It is an important topic, and one of increasing importance as the years go by and life expectancy increases.

Dr. Sapp's writings sparked me to take an interest in the subject. I have been an active Board member of the Alzheimer's Community Care organization in Palm Beach and Martin Counties, Florida. There I see first hand the concern for those who have the disease and the impact it has on those who care for them, and the help needed by both.

Under our Executive Director Mary M. Barnes and her staff, ACC sponsors seven day-care locations from Boca

Raton to Stuart. We provide family consultants to count-less families and individuals in the area. We offer Educational and Training Centers, where more than 1,000 caregivers, professional and others received Dementia Specific Education. The work is never-ending. Across the country other organizations with similar goals also do their marvelous work.

We are sure that Dr. Sapp's book will be helpful to all of those who are involved in any way with Alzheimer's. God bless him, and God bless each of you who cares!

Richard M. Cromie, President
Desert Ministries, Inc.
Palm Beach, Florida

TABLE OF CONTENTS

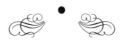

INTRODUCTION

This book is addressed to those who have primary responsibility for the care of a loved one with Alzheimer's disease[1] or a related dementia, and to those who assist such persons. It will also be helpful to family members who are not involved in day-to-day caregiving and to others who want to understand more about the illness and its impact on caregivers. Clergy who would like to minister more effectively to families affected by Alzheimer's disease and friends who want to help but are uncomfortable in the presence of a dementing illness will also benefit. This book thus fits the goal of Desert Ministries: to bring the living water of the Gospel to those in need.

I am grateful to Desert Ministries for the opportunity to revise this book once again, and especially for making available the resources to expand it. As in so many other areas of biomedicine, research and improved practice in the area of dementia proceed apace, and I am confident that progress will continue to be made until a cure is available. Until that wonderful day, I hope this book will make the awesome task of caring for someone with dementia a little more manageable.

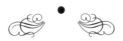

WHEN ALZHEIMER'S DISEASE STRIKES

We all must age and die. Of that, Scripture leaves no doubt: "For everything there is a season, and a time for every matter under heaven: a time to be born, and a time to die" (Ecclesiastes 3:1-2); "The years of our life are threescore and ten, or even by reason of strength fourscore" (Psalm 90:10); "Just as it is appointed for mortals to die once . . ." (Hebrews 9:27). Even when we are able to face up to the inescapable fact of our mortality and accept it for ourselves and our loved ones, we probably imagine (or at least hope) that we and they will die in a relatively quick and painless fashion, in full possession of our faculties as we bravely bid adieu to those we love who have gathered around our bed. Unfortunately, for the increasing number of people in our aging society who suffer from Alzheimer's disease and other dementias, these hopes are far from realized.

The "disease of the century" was the label given to Alzheimer's disease and related forms of senile dementia in 1981 by the late Lewis Thomas, chancellor of Memorial Sloan-Kettering Cancer Center and award-winning essayist. Although a case can be made that AIDS has become the more rightful claimant to that title, no one who has confronted a dementing illness will deny that it is particularly tragic and painful, exacting a heavy toll not only from the person with the disease but from his or her family as well. Indeed, *Time* magazine has called Alzheimer's "the aging brain's most heartbreaking disorder" (July 17, 2000).

Many illnesses deprive a person only of the *present*. One becomes ill, feels more or less miserable depending upon the nature and severity of the illness, seeks treatment, and recovers after a relatively brief period of time, suffering the loss only of that time when one was actually ill. Other illnesses for which no cure exists take away not only a person's present but also the *future* by prematurely ending the individual's life. Alzheimer's disease, however, robs people not only of the present and the future but also of the *past* as their memory of prior events, relationships, and persons gradually slips away.

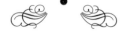

HOW BIG A PROBLEM IS ALZHEIMER'S DISEASE?

According to the latest estimates, approximately four million people in the United States suffer from Alzheimer's disease. If we assume that each of these has four close family members (spouse, children, siblings), the disease actually affects some 20 million people directly, and this number does not include friends who may feel deeply for the person and his or her family. In fact, a survey in the early 1990s found that 37 million Americans said they knew someone with Alzheimer's. When Alzheimer's disease strikes a member of a religious congregation, the number of caring people touched by the illness is likely to increase even more.

These numbers are striking enough, but a glance at the shifting age patterns of the United States population as a whole prompts even deeper concern. From about 4 percent of the population at the beginning of the 20th century, the number of Americans 65 and older grew to around 14 percent by its close—from 3 million to almost 40 million (more than the entire population of Canada!). When the Baby Boomers (the 76 million Americans born between 1946 and 1964, who make up slightly more than one-quarter of the current U.S.

population) start reaching 65 in 2011, the number of older Americans will surge even more markedly, growing to as many as perhaps 70 million or more by 2040, almost 25 percent of the projected total population. The fastest-growing segment of the United States population already comprises those 85 and older, who are 10 percent of the older population today but are expected to reach 20 million and make up as much as 30 percent of all elderly by the middle of this century. Moving even farther along the life span, the number of centenarians in this country quintupled to almost 70,000 between 1980 and today, doubling in the 1990s alone. By 2050 the U.S. Census Bureau projects that as many as 1.1 million people in this country are likely to be over 100!

Why are these numbers so significant? Carl Eisdorfer, an internationally recognized geriatric psychiatrist and one of the founders of the organization now known as the Alzheimer's Association, estimates that the need for care doubles every 5 years a person lives past 65. A sizable portion of that care goes to those suffering from Alzheimer's disease and other dementias because the illness affects primarily older people, although there is a rare form called "early-onset Alzheimer's" that occurs in only five to ten percent of all cases, in which symptoms begin to appear as early as 40. The incidence of Alzheimer's disease also doubles every 5 years beyond 65. Indeed, the 1-in-10 likelihood of developing Alzheimer's at 65 may be as high as 1 in 5 by the time a person reaches 75 and nearly 1 in 2 by age 85 (and remember that those over 85 constitute the most rapidly growing segment of our population). These facts have led experts to estimate that without the cure for which we are all fervently praying, the number of people with Alzheimer's in the United States will approach 6 million by the end of this decade and 14 million by the middle of the century.

Many religious congregations have an even higher percentage of older members than the population in general. For example, 67 percent of the members of the Presbyterian Church (USA) are over the age of 45, 57 percent are over 50, and 35 percent are 65 or older. The median age[2] of members is 54, whereas the median age for the U.S. population as a whole is about 36. This is a trend that is seen across other such denominations, with most reporting that at least 20 to 25 percent of their members are 65 and older. Thus it is especially critical that clergy and laypeople of all faiths learn as much as they can about Alzheimer's disease.

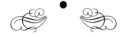

᥆᥆ WHAT IS ALZHEIMER'S DISEASE? ᥆᥆

Alzheimer's disease is precisely that—a disease with its own distinctive effect on a person's body and behavior. Named after the German neuropathologist who in 1906 first described the changes the illness causes in a person's brain, Alzheimer's disease is a progressive, irreversible, degenerative illness that destroys the brain, leading to a condition known as "dementia."

Alzheimer's disease is the most common form of dementia occurring in the U.S. today. *Dementia* means literally "out of one's mind," but the term has a special medical usage: It does not mean "crazy" in normal parlance but rather denotes a loss or impairment of mental capacity serious enough to affect a person's ability to function normally. The condition is marked by specific symptoms that distinguish it clearly, which will be described below. Although a number of dementias exist (not all associated with aging), this book will concentrate on Alzheimer's disease, which comprises the vast majority of cases. Most of what will be said, however, applies with minor variations to the other dementias.

Let me make a very important point here, one that must be clearly understood: Alzheimer's disease and related dementias are not the result of simply "getting old," as some people have come to fear, though the incidence does rise with age. Nor are they in any sense "normal" aging. In fact, if anyone you know begins to demonstrate the symptoms described below, that person should have immediate medical attention, regardless of age. It is an extremely dangerous though still widespread myth that growing older automatically leads to what used to be called "senility," which is often attributed to "hardening of the arteries." It is very important to remember that some 20 to 30 percent of dementias are caused by treatable conditions (e.g., depression, dehydration, malnutrition, infection, or problems with prescription medication), and thus they are partially or completely reversible. Therefore if a loved one of any age begins to show signs of confusion and/or memory loss, get him or her to a competent physician for testing and diagnosis at once.

Despite major advances in Alzheimer's disease research, the cause of the illness remains unknown. A number of theories have been advanced and are constantly being tested. Researchers are closer than ever before to identifying what in all likelihood will turn out to be not *the* cause of Alzheimer's but many *factors* that together contribute to the appearance of the disease. The ones currently considered to be the most likely are *genetic* (you will hear quite a bit about the "APOE gene"), *environmental* (such as head trauma at any age, even much earlier in life), and what I will call "*internal*" (increases in free radicals in the brain, high blood cholesterol levels, high blood pressure and heart disease, and the like).

A recent development that is somewhat confusing merits mention here in passing. In the late 1990s, researchers and physicians began to diagnose and discuss *mild cognitive impairment* (MCI), which some authorities now suggest may be a

8

precursor to Alzheimer's disease (although others argue it is simply very early Alzheimer's). In this condition, the person has persistent memory problems. MCI differs from normal age-related memory change, however, in that the loss is greater than expected, and from Alzheimer's in that the person with MCI does not exhibit other losses typical of dementia, such as confusion, problems with attention, and language difficulties.

Some experts estimate that more than 80 percent of people with mild cognitive impairment develop Alzheimer's disease within 10 years at a rate of 10-15 percent of them a year. This has led to the conclusion that MCI is really early Alzheimer's disease, rather than a separate, distinct condition. Whatever the outcome of this debate, the concept of MCI is important because it has led to studies designed to learn if early diagnosis and treatment can prevent or slow further memory loss, including the development of Alzheimer's disease. You may want to keep your eyes and ears open for more information about this matter, especially if the person you are caring for is in the early stages of Alzheimer's.

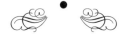

⟨⧓⟩ What Are the Symptoms? ⟨⧓⟩

Although the symptoms of dementia are fairly obvious, they occur in different degrees of severity and varying order of appearance. Early on, many people become quite adept at hiding them, or at least explaining them away. We all misplace keys or eyeglasses, for example. Thus a 75-year-old who does so routinely and laughs off such behavior as "just getting old" seems normal enough (as someone once put it, though, "Don't be too concerned if you forget where you put your keys or glasses—everybody does that. It's time to begin worrying when you can't remember what to do with them when you find them!"). Family members often do not realize something is really wrong until the person cannot find the way to or from a place visited every day or forgets a favorite grandson's visit the previous day.

Probably the best view to take on the question of what is going to happen during the course of Alzheimer's disease is the sage advice that newcomers to family support groups often hear from the "veterans": "When you've seen one Alzheimer's patient . . . you've seen one Alzheimer's patient!" In short, there is simply no such thing as *the* person with Alzheimer's disease. Manifestations of the illness change as it progresses, and thus its impact on caregivers changes also. Generalizations do not necessarily apply to all cases. Just as God made each of us unique, it seems this uniqueness continues to express itself through the early and middle stages of Alzheimer's disease.

Granted that no perfect profile can be drawn of the person suffering from Alzheimer's disease, what *can* be said about the symptoms of the illness? One of the most apt descriptions of Alzheimer's disease is offered by Barry Reisberg, who calls it simply "brain failure," analogous to heart or kidney failure.[3] When one considers the role the brain plays, it is not surprising that virtually every aspect of a person's being and life is significantly affected for the worse by the failure of the organ that controls it all.

Another helpful way to summarize the effect of dementia is to say that it turns the mind into a "cognitive sieve"[4] that is unable to retain the information necessary to function in the world. This tragic situation leads to perhaps the most painful result of Alzheimer's disease for the sufferer and his or her family—namely, the loss of the awareness of oneself as the brain gradually fails to do its normal job.

The earliest manifestation of Alzheimer's disease is usually memory loss, a fact often recalled by caregivers only after the symptoms have become considerably more noticeable. Some minor problems with memory are not unusual as a healthy person ages, but they are temporary and not progressive. In Alzheimer's disease, however, the deterioration of memory continues, normally affecting short-term memory first. Although the person may be able to recall events that occurred decades earlier, yesterday ceases to exist, and five minutes ago may be only a blur. This results from the fact that in its early stages Alzheimer's attacks nerve cells in the hippocampus, the part of the brain that helps us store recent memories. As the disease progresses so does loss of memory, until the person is unable to recognize or name a spouse or sibling.

Associated with short-term memory loss is an increasing inability to learn even the simplest facts and tasks. Although early in the progression of the disease, ways of coping with various losses may be acquired (such as careful note-taking or list-making), this ability is gradually lost as well. Caregivers often become frustrated when they devise ingenious methods that enable the cognitively impaired person to compensate for various lost skills and knowledge, but the person cannot learn even these simple techniques.

Another early manifestation of Alzheimer's disease is difficulty with language (*aphasia*). In the beginning this may appear as use of the wrong word or inability to find the right word. But the capacity to express oneself gradually deteriorates until the person is unable to express him- or herself at all, even with gestures, and cannot relay such basic needs as thirst or a full bladder.

To make matters worse, accompanying this so-called *expressive* aphasia is *receptive* aphasia, that is, the person's inability to understand communications directed to him or her. Thus the simplest explanations must be repeated several times, and even then they may not be "processed" into an appropriate response.

Another symptom that may be connected to memory impairment is loss of the ability to perform various actions and movements essential to functioning independently (*apraxia*). Even the activities of daily living (ADLs) that most people take for granted—such as eating, toileting, bathing, cooking, and cleaning—become increasingly difficult until they can no longer be accomplished at all. Coordination fails, leading from clumsiness to falls to a bedridden state as the brain is progressively unable to direct the body's actions in a purposeful manner. At some point in this process, incontinence will become a problem, creating special difficulties for both the affected person and the caregiver.

Understandably, the person with the illness may undergo significant personality changes and mood swings as the brain is gradually destroyed. The cultured graduate of a finishing school may begin cursing like a sailor and show no concern for appearance or personal hygiene. The tender, caring husband may suddenly become abusive and violent. Aggressive, violent behavior is one of the worst manifestations of this particular class of symptoms, especially when the patient is male and the caregiver female, often old and frail herself. Please be aware, though, that such behavior is far from universal, and your loved one may never exhibit it.

People suffering from a dementing illness often experience disorientation to place and time, especially in unfamiliar settings. This becomes more marked as the disease progresses. Inability to recall the day, date, or even year is common. The person may become increasingly unaware of where he or she is, frequently thinking the present surroundings are a house inhabited many homes ago, or even a childhood home. Needless to say, this problem (compounded by the loss of judgment to be discussed next) often leads to inappropriate behavior, such as mistaking someone for another person, talking too loudly, or even undressing in public.

Yet another result of the destruction of the brain wrought by Alzheimer's disease is loss of judgment. This may be attributable in part to some of the losses already discussed, all of which in turn result from the illness's progression into the cerebral cortex where "higher" mental functions such as language and reasoning are carried out. Although the person with the illness may be able to perform actions such as getting dressed or lighting a stove, he or she may wear a short-sleeved shirt in freezing weather or fail to turn off the gas. One of the biggest problems for caregivers in this regard has to do with driving, when the cognitively impaired person is perfectly capable of performing the *actions* necessary to drive the car but the *judgment* needed to do so safely is lost, along with the memory of *how* to get somewhere or even of *where* one is trying to go.

Another characteristic symptom of Alzheimer's disease as it progresses is the presence of hallucinations and delusions, which often lead to suspicion and paranoia. A woman I knew with Alzheimer's disease was convinced that men were on her patio looking through her windows, and nothing her husband tried could get her to undress and take a bath. Caregivers may be accused of stealing or hiding things, or even of trying to poison the patient. In relating the story of her mother, one caregiver said, "They think everyone is out to get them and their possessions. So they hide everything in the most intricate places and in the most interesting ways, which of course they forget and never find again. I remember my mother's Social Security check was missing for about two weeks until I found it in her underwear drawer, wrapped in a paper towel, plastic wrap, and tied with a string in a nice little bundle. Thank God for direct deposit!"

Among the most troublesome symptoms of dementia for family caregivers are agitation, restlessness, and wandering, which are frequently associated with a disrupted sleep cycle. Some manifestations of these behavior patterns may merely be maddening to the caregiver, such as when the person with

Alzheimer's disease paces from room to room (often in late afternoon and evening in a common phenomenon known as "sundowning"), constantly picks at his or her sweater, or arises and dresses only an hour or two after having been helped to bed at night, thinking it is time to start a new day. The person's tendency to wander away from home, however, oblivious to traffic or the danger of falling or getting lost, is more than a nuisance. A daughter recalls, "At the beginning of my mother's illness, she would take off for a walk while I was at work. My 12-year-old son had to chase my mother down the street on his bicycle to make sure she would come back home." This common behavior obviously poses a genuine threat to the safety of the individual, especially if the person has begun to show some of the other symptoms like loss of judgment, difficulty walking, or poor perception.

How Is Alzheimer's Disease Diagnosed?

Because the cause of Alzheimer's is unknown, no simple procedure exists to demonstrate definitively whether or not a person has the disease (unlike, say, pneumonia, where a culture can positively identify the germ that is causing it). At this time, the only way to get an absolutely certain diagnosis is through microscopic examination of brain tissue after death. The pathologist looks to see if certain regions of the brain contain abnormal deposits of the protein beta-amyloid and collections of twisted fibers inside nerve cells—the "amyloid plaques and neurofibrillary tangles" long known to be characteristic of Alzheimer's.[5]

So for people who are showing symptoms of dementia like confusion and difficulty with memory, physicians must make a diagnosis of "possible" or "probable" Alzheimer's disease by ruling out other medical problems that can cause similar symptoms. If the results of all the tests described below fit the pattern of Alzheimer's, the diagnosis will be "probable Alzheimer's disease." If the results are not completely typical of Alzheimer's but nothing else is found to be causing them, the diagnosis will be "possible Alzheimer's disease."

The diagnostic process consists of a number of steps, beginning with the all-important medical history. This should be as thorough as possible, taking special note of other family members who may have exhibited signs of dementia (about 1 in 10 people with Alzheimer's has a parent or sibling similarly afflicted). A complete physical examination is essential as well and will include a battery of blood tests, a urine test, a standard neurological exam, and perhaps various brain imaging procedures, such as computed tomography (CT) or the more effective magnetic resonance imaging (MRI), positron emission tomography (PET), and single photon emission computed tomography (SPECT). The first two techniques reveal changes in the brain tissue itself, which can be helpful because early in the development of Alzheimer's disease certain parts of the brain, such as the hippocampus, shrink. These tests can also detect other possible causes of dementia symptoms like stroke or tumor. The other two imaging techniques detect abnormalities in the actual functioning of the brain by depicting the response of various parts of the brain to different activities or by showing the pattern of blood circulation in the brain.

Not surprisingly, a very thorough psychological ("mental status") examination will be conducted. This consists of several tests that have been shown to detect problems typical of Alzheimer's and to rule out other causes of some symptoms, for example, depression. Answers to instructions and questions such as "Count backward from 20 to 1," "Say the months in reverse order," "What day is today?" and "Who is the President of the United States?" provide a good indication of the person's reasoning capability, orientation to time, and memory. The ability to carry out activities of daily living and normal social interactions is also assessed.

Such a thorough evaluation involves a number of different specialists and is expensive, time-consuming, and tiring. If the person with dementia has advanced to a certain point in the illness, the experience can be difficult for both the person and the caregiver, who must normally be present to offer assistance of various kinds. Unfortunately, this is often the case because family members are usually loath to acknowledge what is happening to their loved one and many physicians are not very aware of the early signs.

Understanding many of the procedures and terminology involved is often overwhelming for family members who are deeply concerned about the loved one being evaluated, not to mention for the person being put through the ordeal. Do not be afraid or embarrassed to ask the physicians and others involved in the evaluation to explain everything as clearly and thoroughly as possible. You need to be comfortable with what is happening and with what you are told, and you have a right to know—as does your loved one if he or she is able to understand.

CAN ALZHEIMER'S DISEASE BE CURED OR TREATED?

Despite the complexity and difficulty of diagnosis, physicians who are experienced in dealing with dementia will make a correct diagnosis in eight or nine of every 10 cases.[6] Even if a relatively definitive diagnosis can been made, however, it is important for families of people with Alzheimer's to recognize that at the current level of medical knowledge, no effective long-term treatment for the disease or even for most of its symptoms exists. This is not to say that many of the problems it causes cannot be managed. Still, although we know a great deal more about Alzheimer's disease than ever before, the discovery of the cause or a cure is not yet on the horizon. Some researchers even suspect that Alzheimer's may well be not a single disease with a single cause but a multiplicity of diseases with a variety of causes, some genetic and some environmental. In fact, genetic research in particular is beginning to yield some hopeful results.

A great deal of research on drugs for Alzheimer's has been carried out in recent years, and although some progress has occurred, families often get their hopes up only to have them dashed. In the summer of 1999, the media trumpeted reports of AN-1792, a vaccine that showed great promise in animal tests not only in preventing the disease but also in reversing damage that had already occurred. The success of a small-scale study to test the drug's safety in humans gave many people even greater hope. Unfortunately, 15 of the participants in the next level of testing (to determine proper dosages) developed severe brain inflammation, and the manufacturer closed the study permanently on March 1, 2002.

Today, only four drugs are approved by the Food and Drug Administration (FDA) for the treatment of Alzheimer's disease: Cognex—announced in 1993 with considerable publicity and overstated claims—has shown limited effectiveness and only in the early stages of Alzheimer's. It is rarely prescribed because of negative side effects and the need to take several doses a day. Aricept (1996), the drug most often prescribed today, is effective in moderating symptoms in some people, but only for a maximum of about two years. Exelon (2000) and Reminyl (2001) offer improvement in day-to-day functioning, behavior, and mental activities such as thinking, reasoning, and speaking for those with mild-to-moderate symptoms. Although these drugs cannot stop or reverse the progression of Alzheimer's disease, they can slow the rate of decline and improve quality of life. For the benefit of your loved one and yourself, take time to have a serious conversation with the doctor about these drugs and others as they become available in the future.

A number of other possible treatments for Alzheimer's disease or ways to prevent it are under formal study[7] or are simply being touted by proponents as effective with little or no scientific evidence for such claims. These include vitamin E, which shows possible moderate functional improvement in early- to mid-stage Alzheimer's; estrogen replacement therapy, which has some evidence for lower risk of developing the disease and improved cognition but is not without risk; anti-inflammatory agents (NSAIDs such as naproxen and ibuprofen and COX-2 inhibitors such as Celebrex and Vioxx),which show possible delay of Alzheimer's onset if used regularly but again can be dangerous if not used carefully; lipid-lowering agents (statins), which lower cholesterol levels and in doing so perhaps reduce the risk of Alzheimer's disease; gamma- and beta-secretase inhibitors, which block the production of a protein in the brain associated with Alzheimer's; and gingko biloba, although there is no compelling evidence of its effectiveness in treating Alzheimer's.

It is beyond the scope of this book to discuss in detail these possible treatments and preventive measures (or others that may have their "30 seconds of fame"). By all means, though, you should keep abreast of the latest research in any way you can. Ask your physician what is going on, and insist on more than a cursory dismissal if you have heard about something that sounds promising. The Internet is an excellent way to gather a great deal of information quickly, but remember to check the validity of the sources! And definitely give prayerful considera-tion to participating in clinical trials of new drugs if your loved one is an acceptable candidate. At the very least you will be helping others by doing so, thereby fulfilling the central com-mandment of both Judaism and Christianity that we should love and serve others, even if there is no reward in it for us.[8]

Be very cautious, however, of anyone who promises a "mir-acle cure" or guarantees successful treatment, especially in return for a large amount of money. Such a cure simply does not exist. In their desperation, Alzheimer's caregivers can easily fall prey to unscrupulous and uncaring people. If you find yourself tempted to pursue such a possibility, please discuss the matter with your loved one's regular physician before committing your resources. He or she should know the facts and the true effectiveness of any proposed treatment.

Earlier, I mentioned AIDS as a legitimate contender with Alzheimer's for the title "disease of the century" (whether the 20th or the 21st). There is another connection between the two illnesses that can be noted in this context: Immense strides have been made in understanding AIDS and the human immunodeficiency virus (HIV) that causes it, which are leading to considerable progress in the development of treatments that can delay the devastating and invariably fatal effects of the illness. So far, however, no one claims to be close to an actual cure. Similarly, we have noted a number of recent advances in Alzheimer's research and the promise of even more. These are leading to equally great improvements in treating various aspects of the disease, or at least in managing its symptoms and slowing its progress somewhat. Most authorities, however, do not anticipate that anyone is on the verge of a discovery that will sound the death knell for Alzheimer's disease itself.

I would like to make a suggestion to all those affected by this disease who want to strike a real blow at dementia and offer hope to people affected by it. As we have seen, despite significant progress, a great deal of research lies ahead before Alzheimer's disease falls into the same category as, say, heart disease—that is, an illness that is potentially deadly, but for which effective prevention and treatment strategies exist. Becoming an *advocate for increased research funding for Alzheimer's* would be a tremendous service with an impact far beyond that which any individual could make, especially as the 76 million baby boomers begin to approach the age of increasing susceptibility.

An increase in research would also be a wise investment for an aging society because, apart from the personal costs that are the focus of this book, the economic cost of Alzheimer's disease is staggering. Dr. Robert N. Butler, the first director of the National Institute on Aging, has pointed out that we are already spending as much as $100 billion a year in care related to Alzheimer's disease. By the time the Baby Boomers reach retirement age, as many as 9 million people in the U.S. will have the illness, more than double the number today.

With rising life expectancy and the increased incidence of Alzheimer's as one gets older, delaying the onset of the disease only five years would mean that one-half of those who would otherwise exhibit significant symptoms of the disease would die of natural causes before becoming disabled by it. Thus those who can become active and vocal about the need for more research funding—particularly those who can speak from first-hand experience about the problems that Alzheimer's disease brings to families—can provide a tremendous service to many, many people and bring hope to those who may be concerned about what the future holds for them in terms of developing this illness.

In summary, it needs to be said again that Alzheimer's disease is "brain failure." We are not surprised when a person with heart failure is unable to spend the afternoon on a vigorous hike in the woods. Just so, we should hardly be surprised at any behaviors caused by losing the organ that is responsible not only for the physical functioning of the human body but also for personality and emotions as well. It is therefore critically important to keep in mind that just as we do not *blame* a person with heart disease for the inability to engage in vigorous exercise, we cannot blame the person with "brain disease" for his or her behavior, however bizarre, inappropriate, or seemingly inexplicable it is.

What Does Alzheimer's Disease Do to a Family?

Recall the numbers I cited earlier about the aging population of the United States and the increasing incidence of Alzheimer's disease associated with it. Now realize that more than 70 percent of people with Alzheimer's disease live at home, and about 75 percent of these receive their care from family and friends. The other 25 percent is paid care that costs an average of $12,500 per year, almost all of which is paid out-of-pocket by the families. Clearly, the impact of caring for those with Alzheimer's disease falls most heavily on family members. And it is a heavy burden, to be sure.

Indeed, unlike with most other illnesses, with Alzheimer's the entire *family* has the disease, or feels as if it has. You cannot allow yourself to feel guilty if you have come to the end of your rope both physically and emotionally, because it cannot be denied that family members who care for persons with dementia are also victims of the disease.

Just as there is great variability in the course of the illness and in the effect it has on the individual with dementia, families' reactions to the stress of caring for a cognitively impaired person vary greatly. Nonetheless, certain reactions seem to be fairly common, and people who provide constant care to someone who is gradually deteriorating mentally as well as physically need to know what to expect. Of course, the effects of dementia on a family discussed here are by no means all that may occur, and many of them interact and overlap.

• • •

⤫ ROLE CHANGES ⤫

When Alzheimer's disease strikes, one of the most difficult problems for families is the role changes that inevitably occur. If the caregiver is the spouse, he or she must often assume not just new *responsibilities*—such as cooking, laundry, keeping the checkbook, and so forth—but also the new *role* that accompanies such changes. For example, the husband may have been the decision-maker for the family in terms of major purchases, vacation plans, or evenings out. Now, unable to subtract 3 from 20 or button his own shirt, he must relinquish control to a wife who has always been happy to follow his lead. Or the wife may have handled all the domestic tasks from cooking and cleaning to paying the bills, and suddenly at the age of 70, her husband must assume these responsibilities. Such a radical reorientation in patterns of living that have developed over decades is extremely difficult for everybody involved.

The situation may be even worse if an adult child is the primary caregiver. Most people never get over the deep-seated feeling that one's parent is one's parent, and there is something very difficult in having the person who was once the "adult" gradually become the "child." One caregiving daughter gave voice to it this way: "Becoming my mother's mother was *not* what I had in mind at this time in my life!" Very few people are comfortable assuming the parental role for their own mother or father, especially when personal care such as dressing, toileting, and bathing becomes a necessity, and particularly when the parent is the opposite sex.

Of course, this role reversal causes significant problems for the parent who is still aware of what is going on because—in addition to the loss of independence and self-determination it demonstrates—one of the most difficult developmental tasks we face as parents is learning to see our children as adults. If parents have never learned to accept that their children have "grown up," at the time the children must have more input into the parents' lives and assume more control over them, a great deal of tension, discomfort, and pain inevitably result. Perhaps it would be wise (and valuable in ways far beyond this context) for all parents to make more of an effort to accept their children's adult status.

If the child and parent have not had a particularly good relationship, of course, the situation is even worse, and the resentment at having to give up one's own life to care for a parent one has never particularly cared for can be great. In such cases, some serious thought needs to be given (perhaps in consultation with one's clergyperson) to the meaning of the Fifth Commandment, "Honor your father and your mother" (Exodus 20:12).[9] If, however, the situation is truly intolerable for all parties, the best way to "honor" a demented parent may be to put that person in a situation where good care is available without the pain and stress caused by a difficult parent-child relationship.

Conflicts among siblings can also arise when care decisions

about parents must be made. These tensions may result from unresolved childhood issues ("Mom always liked you better!"), or simply because different people have different values and different ideas about how things should be done. Maybe the child who has been the stable, mature sibling lives far from the ill parent, and the "baby" of the family—the child everyone has always made excuses for or dismissed as hopelessly immature and irresponsible—is now thrust into the role of primary caregiver.

The situation becomes even more complicated when an elderly spouse is the primary caregiver but an adult child is on the scene to "offer advice." For some reason, as our parents age we tend to begin to feel that they cannot make decisions as well as we can, even when those decisions concern their own lives. We feel that their judgment is flawed and that we know better. Caregiving spouses often report conflict with adult children who do not understand what it is like to live 24 hours a day with a demented person and who think things should be done differently.

The same problem can arise among siblings, especially when one is the primary caregiver and the others only "check in" occasionally. Often the person actually providing the care feels unfairly dumped on, even when willing to accept the responsibility. Resentment easily arises when absentee siblings question or criticize the care being given, or even when they make innocent suggestions or raise important issues in good faith. An excellent illustration of this problem is a remark made by a woman at a support group meeting. After talking about the difficulties of being the on-the-scene caregiver with siblings scattered across the country "advising" her on their mother's care, she said, "If there's such a thing as reincarnation, I've decided I want to come back in my next life as the 'sister from out of town.'"

Incidentally, this comment also illustrates one of the most effective coping devices available to an Alzheimer's caregiver, one that every caregiver should strive to utilize if at all possible, namely, humor. A piece of advice frequently given to support group newcomers by the "Alzheimer's old-timers" is that you must have a sense of humor to survive the ordeal. As one veteran caregiver put it, "You *have* to laugh; you can't cry all the time." Of course, your sense of humor must be displayed appropriately and with care. But sometimes the only way to respond to something a person with Alzheimer's says or does is with good cheer and a smile. This, by the way, can also have a beneficial effect on the person, who will often respond positively to the smile or laughter, even with no understanding of what prompted it.

Appropriate humor can often help diffuse tension and conflict within a family as well. A more effective approach, however, is to hold a conference to air your problems and to work on resolving them. The advice that God gave the people of Judah through the prophet Isaiah is still valid: "Come now, let us reason together" (1:18). Your minister can be an excellent person to help with this project. Most clergy have education and experience that will allow them to maintain order while providing an objective, trained ear to help sort through the underlying issues, which may not be recognized by the participants because of their emotional investments and decades-old patterns of relating to one another. The minister can identify points of conflict and avenues of resolution that family members could never discover on their own. Remember, too, that such family negotiations will likely need to be an ongoing process because as the disease progresses, changes will occur in the dynamics of caregiving, and decisions will have to be made and revised regularly.

• • •

∾ GRIEF ∾

Overarching the problems occasioned by role changes is a deep sense of *loss* that everyone involved in the situation feels. This leads to grief. With a dementing illness, however, grief is somewhat different the experienced in most other situations. After watching her husband deteriorate over the years, one caregiver offered the now well-known description that it was like "the funeral that never ends." Little by little, personality trait by personality trait, expression by expression, a loved one fades away. A spouse will eventually realize that the partner with whom he or she has spent decades is gone. Yet physically the person may still be quite robust and will certainly be demanding. An adult child caregiver must come to grips with the fact that the parent who has symbolized security and wisdom has slowly become like a child again. The sense of loss and loneliness, the stark realization that the person you have always counted on and leaned on in tough times is gradually slipping away, can be overwhelming.

Constant interaction with a person with Alzheimer's also forces caregiving spouses (and perhaps especially children and grandchildren) to acknowledge their own aging. This is another sense of loss that can be particularly painful if a person has never confronted his or her mortality before. We do not view aging in a positive light, and Alzheimer's disease is one of the most discouraging examples of aging imaginable. When in my Religious Issues in Death and Dying class the high incidence of Alzheimer's disease in people over 85 was mentioned, one of my 21-year-old senior students immediately responded, "I'm going to die before I get that old." When I asked her if she was serious or just being flip, she said, looking me directly in the eyes with no hint of a smile on her face, "I'm completely serious."[10] Virtually all of the world's major religions, however, affirm the importance, even the necessity, of acknowledging one's mortality if one is to find true spiritual maturity.[11] Therefore being made aware of one's mortality by caring for a person with Alzheimer's disease should not be seen in a totally negative light.

Nonetheless, for the person who is experiencing this confrontation with mortality at the same time that she or he is facing the myriad problems of caring for a cognitively impaired relative, the opportunity for spiritual growth may not be appreciated. If I am speaking to you, ask your clergyperson to help you work through this important issue.

Eventually, of course, the physical death of the person must be faced. Despite the opportunity for "anticipatory grief" that dementia provides family members—not to mention the relief that is inevitably mingled with pain—the actual death is still difficult. One caregiver said that she grieved twice: once when her mother entered a nursing home (for the person her mother had been) and again when her mother died (for the sweet, confused woman she had become).

The final stages of the disease are not pleasant. Caregivers are usually exhausted physically, mentally, emotionally, and often financially. They need to find a way to discuss their mixed feelings about the death, especially the often-expressed wish that the person die rather than continue to suffer such indignity and even—in many people's eyes—dehumanization. It is also very common to wrestle with the almost unavoidable feeling that the person's death will come as a welcome relief from the burden of caregiving (see the next section for more on this issue). In addition, it is essential that all those involved in the person's life explore in advance their feelings about the difficult choices that attend death in a chronic illness, such as withholding or withdrawing life-sustaining treatment (including food and water),[12] so that sound decisions can be made if such a situation arises.

• • •

∝ GUILT ∝

The preceding discussion suggests one of the most difficult problems that family caregivers face, one about which our religious traditions have a great deal to say, namely, guilt. Caregivers often express feelings of guilt that they have contributed to the loved one's contracting the illness, or that they sometimes wish the person would die, or especially that they should be able to do more than they are. It is a source of constant amazement to professionals who work with caregivers to listen to them describe a level of dedication, commitment, tolerance, and sheer physical exertion that is exhausting just to hear about, only to have them conclude, "I feel so guilty that I'm not doing more" or "that I couldn't figure out what he wanted."

One woman in a support group summarized a new participant's expression of such feelings by saying, "Guilt, guilt, guilt—we all have it!" Another commented, "I think the 'G-word' gives caregivers more trouble than anything else." If you suffer from feelings of guilt, a good piece of advice is to realize that it is impossible for anybody to carry out the caregiver's responsibilities. So simply do the best you can.

Such guilt often appears completely irrational to an outsider. A caregiver may feel guilty for wanting to get away alone for a little while, make a phone call, or just go to the bathroom without interruption. Sometimes people feel that they are responsible for a decline in the person's condition (or for the disease itself), or that their situation is punishment for not caring enough for the person before the illness. Another support group member voiced the guilt that comes from the collision of religious values with the difficult necessities of caregiving when she said, "I have this Christian guilt trip about lying to my mother when I hide her purse so she won't try to go out, and then when she asks me if I know where it is, I say 'no.'"

There is also the more legitimate guilt that results from the unavoidable anger caregivers often feel. This anger sometimes leads to verbal or physical abuse of the demented person. Indeed, abuse of the elderly (and not only of those with dementia) is a growing problem in our society. It is often very difficult not to react to someone's diminishing cognitive capacities and physical abilities with sarcastic or sharp comments, even when you are well aware of the hurt this causes and do not want to respond in such a way. If you find yourself becoming abusive to the person for whom you are caring, *please* seek help.

Guilt can be an especially troublesome problem for the caregiver who makes the dangerous (and unwise) promise, "Don't worry; I'll never put you in a nursing home," and then has to do it. Even without such a promise, the guilt caused by having to institutionalize a loved one is often so strong that it delays the decision far beyond the point when it should have been made or interferes with continued caregiving because family members cannot stand to see the person in "that place where we put her."

If such feelings actually prevent visits or reduce their number below that which the caregiver believes to be "right," even more guilt is generated. This then becomes a particularly vicious circle. Also, if a caregiver reaches the point of physical and emotional exhaustion and institutionalization becomes the only alternative, the caregiver may have to deal with the additional guilt from accusations of "putting Dad away" or "getting rid of Mom." These charges often come from relatives who have participated minimally in the care of the cognitively impaired person and perhaps have rarely even visited.

Guilt feelings are a perfectly normal, unavoidable human reaction to the situation in which caregivers often find themselves. But however normal and unavoidable, such feelings are not easy to admit to others or perhaps even to acknowledge to oneself. The negative effects of unresolved guilt for a person's health, however, are well documented, and you must find an approach that allows you to acknowledge your guilt and work toward resolving it. Your clergyperson can be very helpful in this regard.

I have found it helpful for people struggling with this problem to understand the distinction between *guilt*, an objective result of really doing something wrong for which one should feel bad, and a *sense of guilt*, a subjective response that is not necessarily based on any blameworthy behavior.[12] There is, in fact, a great difference between *being* guilty and *feeling* guilty.

Experience suggests that the vast majority of caregiver's guilt is merely a sense of guilt—just as painful perhaps, but certainly not warranted.

• • •

❧ ANGER ❧

In addition to guilt, one of the most constant companions of families with Alzheimer's disease is anger. When you exhaust yourself to help a loved one who forgets five minutes later what you have done, tells a visitor you don't care what happens, or even accuses you of mistreating him or her, the natural reaction is to be angry and hurt, especially if others give credence to such remarks. It is very difficult to live day in and day out, not to mention all night every night, with the bizarre behaviors of a demented person who may appear completely "normal" physically without wanting to shout, "Why are you doing this? Why don't you just stop acting this way?"

The answers to those questions, of course, are that the person has no idea why and cannot stop. Thus anger can be especially painful because at one level you know that the ill person cannot help the irritating behavior, and then you feel guilty for being angry at a "sick person who can't help it." As one caregiver put it, "You know they can't help themselves and they don't know what they're doing, but you still can't help getting angry." Or another: "The mixture of frustration and guilt is overwhelming. Even when one can logically understand that it is not the person's fault to wake up and get dressed 10 times at night, it is frustrating and exhausting. Consequently, this brings me more guilt for feeling angry." If you want to cope successfully, you must keep in mind that the cognitively impaired person's actions are the result of the disease and are not aimed at you personally.

The anger and frustration that you feel are not always directed at the sick person, of course. The disease itself—or perhaps more generally, the whole situation—provokes considerable anger. This was well expressed by a woman whose father died of Alzheimer's disease after four years of deterioration who said, "It's just wrong and grossly unfair that a person's mind can be taken away, especially when you can see it happening right in front of your eyes." Sometimes a couple has dreamed, planned, and worked for years to travel during their retirement, and just as that possibility becomes reality, Alzheimer's disease cruelly strips it away. Anger is a perfectly normal reaction in such a situation, and it is compounded by profound sadness and a deep sense of loss.

You may be angry with other family members for their failure to help out, personally or financially. The doctors and other health care professionals may be the target of some of your hostility—sometimes with reason if they are aloof, uncaring, or lacking knowledge, but more often just because they cannot really do much regardless of how sincere and caring they are.

Of course, God gets a healthy share of anger as well for allowing this to happen to a "wonderful Christian like Joe" or to "someone like Lois who always attended church faithfully" (not to mention to *you* also!). Overlaying this anger is guilt for being angry with God, which is certainly a taboo in most people's minds. I think God understands your anger, however, and I cannot imagine that God wants your burden increased by guilt. Indeed, many Psalms are expressions of anger and disappointment at God for allowing some misfortune to befall the Psalmist, and they are part of sacred Scripture! So unload your feelings, and continue to know that "underneath are the everlasting arms" (Deuteronomy 33:27) that will hold you up even through this time of trial, just as your earthly parents did not cease to love and support you even when as a child you got angry at them.

• • •

∽ HELPLESSNESS AND LOSS OF HOPE ∽

Many caregivers experience a sense of helplessness and loss of hope that things will ever be better: "As her daughter, the worst part of the disease for me was the helplessness of seeing my mother lose her faculties without being able to do anything for her. Seeing her become more depressed each day with the realization of her forgetfulness was devastating for me." Caring for a person with dementia can seem like a never-ending task with little in the way of tangible reward. After all, the person will not get better and often is unable to express any appreciation for what is being done for him or her. And indeed, with Alzheimer's disease there is no hope in the sense that the word is often used in regard to illness. So I do not want to be the vehicle through a Pollyanna attitude for imparting or encouraging unrealistic expectations that can only be disappointing for you in the long run. Such an attitude could even cause you to question your own feelings by making you think that your anger, guilt, frustration, self-pity, and hopelessness are not normal and unavoidable reactions, which I trust you realize by now they most certainly are. Furthermore, if I offered you too much optimism here, I would not blame you for throwing this book away because you *know* what you really are up against, and nothing I can say can change that.

So, as Morrie Schwartz put it so well in the context of his battle with ALS ("Lou Gehrig's Disease"), another invariably degenerative and fatal illness, "Be hopeful but not foolishly hopeful." He went on to say more about what he meant, and though he was speaking as the person who *has* the illness, his words are equally applicable to your situation as a caregiver:

"When you learn you have a serious illness, you naturally hope that it isn't as serious as it appears to be or as you've been told it is. You may have let your hope run away with you, and you find out your expectations are quite unrealistic. On the other hand, you don't want to feel hopeless. It would be folly to think there will be a cure for ALS in time to save me, but to hope that my ALS will reach a plateau or move slowly is realistic. I can be hopeful about continuing to be effective and useful for a while longer."[14]

The world of dementia into which you have been thrust is in many ways a strange one indeed. Nonetheless, opportunities for love, joy, and laughter still exist, and though there is no cure available, there are ways to improve the quality of life for the entire family. Some good things can even result from the experience of being a caregiver (see pages 55-57, "Positive Aspects of Caregiving"). I want you to know and remember this.

In fact, Clare Booth Luce's observation, "There are no hopeless situations, only people who have grown hopeless about them," is particularly applicable to caring for a person with Alzheimer's disease. Certainly the message of the

Christian faith, acknowledging as it does the full reality of the pain and suffering you are experiencing, can be a beacon of hope in the face of despair (remember Jesus on the cross, suffering so terribly that he wondered if God had forsaken him; yet on the other side of the suffering lay the glory of the new life of resurrection). As someone once said, "Hope has to do with the presence of God, not the absence of struggle," an affirmation that calls to mind the words of Dr. Martin Luther King, Jr., "We must accept finite disappointment, but we must never lose infinite hope."

So I urge you to cultivate your relationship with a higher spiritual power, however you conceive it. If you belong to a formal religious organization, allow that group to be a caring, supportive community, perhaps by helping them understand *how* they can be. It may go a long way toward balancing the inevitable feelings of helplessness and hopelessness that accompany dementia.

The best advice that I can offer to those who find themselves caring for a person with Alzheimer's disease may have been given by poet-statesman Vaclav Havel when he said, "Hope is not about believing you can change things. Hope is about believing you make a difference." It is true that you will not be able to change the ultimate outcome of the situation in which you find yourself, but you can take great comfort and satisfaction in the fact that you make a great difference in the life of your loved one!

• • •

⬙ EMBARRASSMENT ⬙

More mundane than hopelessness, but nonetheless very real, is the embarrassment that many families feel. People with dementia engage in a number of behaviors that most people find embarrassing or even offensive. Yet because they appear relatively "normal" physically for so long during the disease, it is easy to feel they are responsible for their actions. They do not have the "presence of mind," however, to modify, apologize for, or even acknowledge their inappropriate behavior. Thus many family members are embarrassed by such behavior and feel obliged to make explanations and apologies or worse, to isolate the person and keep him or her "out of sight." This course of action can contribute to further loss of contact with reality on the patient's part.

It is important to remember that the person is truly not responsible for his or her actions or words, however inappropriate they are. People who comment critically on the patient's strange behavior are hardly worth your concern for their feelings. On the other hand, if you feel up to it, you can consider using these occasions to educate an obviously ignorant person about Alzheimer's disease.

Continuing to take your loved one to religious functions for as long as possible, where your fellow believers can be told openly what the problem is and where you will find love and support, will give you and the ill person an ongoing opportunity to get out and be among people who genuinely care and at least try to understand. Of course, here too you may need to do a little educating of the congregation—maybe even the clergyperson—about the nature of Alzheimer's disease. But it will be a service to them as well as to others in your community who share the burden you bear.

• • •

◆ ISOLATION ◆

Many of the problems discussed above contribute to another difficulty that family caregivers experience, namely, the feeling of isolation, that they must carry the burden alone on a seemingly endless journey. Unfortunately, all too often, what they experience is more than just a *feeling* of isolation. If the caregiver is a spouse, he or she may feel abandoned by husband or wife at precisely the point in their lives when they were expecting to be able to spend quality time together without the obligations and distractions of children and career. If an adult child is the caregiver, he or she may feel disappointed and let down, even deserted, by a parent who can no longer be a source of strength, security, and authority.

Beyond these extremely painful experiences, families stricken with Alzheimer's disease often find that their friends are uncomfortable interacting with someone who is cognitively impaired. When there is no hope for recovery or even improvement on the part of the patient, it can be difficult to know what to say to the caregiver as well. Friends generally support someone who is suffering temporary pain and is making an effort to get well as quickly as possible. But when it becomes apparent that the suffering will go on and on with no chance of recovery, it is not surprising that people tend to avoid such painful situations and stop visiting. Caregivers' feelings of isolation and abandonment are further compounded by the difficulty they have in leaving their impaired relatives and getting out by themselves, a problem that unfortunately increases as the disease progresses.

Ironically, the isolation that many caregivers experience may be made worse by a particularly vexing problem. If there is one thing Americans are known for and take pride in, it is our keen sense of independence, which is virtually an obsession today. Although this excessive emphasis on independence manifests itself in many ways, in the context of caring for a person with dementia it is most evident in the inability of many caregivers to accept help. Whether stemming from a misguided sense of pride or deeply felt self-reliance, it leads to difficulty admitting that they cannot take care of their loved ones completely on their own. Even people who would like to help may be made to feel unwelcome because a caregiver is too proud to acknowledge the need for assistance of any kind, including spiritual support. This attitude can be compounded by the trouble many older people (and some younger ones) have in acknowledging the need for help with what appears to be a "mental" problem. Our society has not yet overcome its longstanding prejudice toward mental illness and a "blame-the-victim" mentality that is not so prevalent with physical ailments such as cancer or stroke.

Of course, it is not surprising that those who have been responsible for meeting virtually all of the ill person's needs come to feel that they can do best whatever must be done. This is probably a legitimate feeling in many cases. A fierce attitude of "I can do it by myself," however, deters offers of help that may still be made and can even hinder the provision of the best care possible by failing to utilize resources that may be available in the family, religious institution, or community. For example, in the early stages of the illness, adult day-care or some form of "respite care" can afford a wonderful opportunity for caregivers to continue some semblance of a life of their own and to have a little time to "recharge their spiritual (and physical) batteries."

It is simply undeniable that years of responsibility for a demented individual can destroy even the strongest and most dedicated person. I want to encourage you to open yourself to offers of assistance and support and even to ask for help when you need it. As Debbie Anderson, director of Senior Health Service at Overlake Hospital in Bellevue, Washington, has so aptly put it, "Real independence is not living without help; it is knowing when to ask for help so you can accomplish what you truly want." Thus it is actually a *sign of strength* to be able to ask for help. Sadly, many caregivers view it as a weakness and send a clear message to everybody that they can manage quite well alone, thank you very much! Then when relatives and friends want to help, they get the impression that their expressions of concern are seen as meddling. Sometimes they go ahead and try anyway, but they are rebuffed.

If you find yourself having trouble asking for help or accepting it when it is offered, remember this profound observation from a caregiver of a person with Alzheimer's: "Even Superman is Clark Kent most of the time!" Instead of trying to do it all yourself, keep a list of people who say, "Let me know if I can help," and when something comes up with which you need assistance, call someone on the list. You can also make a list of things you need help with, and when someone makes a general offer of aid, be prepared to consult your list and say, "Well, actually, I could use your help tomorrow morning in getting Mom to the doctor," or "Can you come over this afternoon and clean the air-conditioner filters because Bert just can't do it anymore?"

One of the very best things you can do to overcome the feeling of isolation is to attend a support group. Support groups are meetings of caregivers, often (and preferably) under the guidance of a person trained in group dynamics and process who can facilitate sharing. Many support groups meet in churches, synagogues, and community centers. Among the benefits that family caregivers report from support groups are help in understanding why the person behaves a certain way and in learning specific and practical ways to deal with particular behaviors; information about the disease, treatment options, and community resources, such as good doctors and day-care programs; permission to acknowledge and express negative or ambivalent feelings; and emotional support, including the realization that others are in the same boat yet are managing to cope.

A long-time member of a support group expressed the value it held for her with only a little exaggeration when she said to a first-time participant, "You will find out more from us than you'll ever learn from the doctors." At the very least, attending such a group will put you in contact with others who will be very empathic and supportive. In turn, such interaction will provide some hope in what may appear to be a hopeless situation when you see that others are coping and surviving.

As I mentioned before, early recognition of Alzheimer's disease is becoming increasingly common. Thus more and more people are being diagnosed while they are still capable of understanding what is happening to them. With the variable course of the disease, many people now live 8 to 20 years after a tentative diagnosis and are often only mildly impaired for a long time. One result is that the first-hand experiences of people with Alzheimer's disease are beginning to be heard in large numbers, and support groups not just for caregivers but also for the persons with Alzheimer's are springing up across the country.

These meetings give people in the early stages of the illness—those who can no longer work, whose friends and business associates have abandoned them, and who perhaps recognize the burden they place on their caregiver—an opportunity to be with others who share these same experiences and feelings and thus can understand them in a way no one else can. Such support groups can help people with Alzheimer's recognize that despite their illness, they still have a life to live, and this realization can inspire them to keep trying rather than give up.

The nature and structure of these groups vary, with some being primarily for socializing, some for sharing tips on ways to cope with problems common to Alzheimer's, and some merely for giving people a forum in which to express their feelings about what is happening to them. Whatever the nature of the group, as with caregivers' groups so support groups for Alzheimer's patients enable participants to realize that they are not alone in suffering the losses they are experiencing. As one man put it, "These days a good day is when I can go to my support group. I have the feeling that life is okay. Nobody's cheering, but at least it's okay."

Let me mention in this context an extremely important fact to keep in mind: For some time, the existence of "learned helplessness" has been recognized in nursing home settings and some family-care situations. This is where caregivers take over more and more of the lives of the people for whom they are caring because it is so much easier to do it themselves than to encourage and assist those who are impaired to do something. Thus those being cared for "learn" to be helpless, and as a result they deteriorate more quickly. The caregiver's goal, however, should be to help the person function at the highest level possible at that time. This is especially important with increasing early diagnosis of the illness. Some people in the very early stages can even continue to do volunteer work or perform long-time household responsibilities, and every effort should be made to encourage them to do so.

This is also a good place to alert you to an essential resource. The Alzheimer's Association is the nationally recognized leader in addressing dementing illnesses. Most large communities have a local chapter that will be able to give you information about the disease and support groups in your area and offer you encouragement and support when you need it. As one caregiver wrote after listing nearly a dozen of the "hardest things" she had had to deal with in that role, "If I didn't have people like those I've met through the Alzheimer's Association, I simply don't think I'd be able to function. When I get into one of my 'Poor me, why is this happening?' moods, I know there is someone there who will listen to me whine and then give me the kick I need to get on with it." For the number and location of your local Alzheimer's Association chapter, call the national office in Chicago at 800-272-3900, log on to www.alz.org, or write to the Alzheimer's Association, 919 North Michigan Avenue, Suite 1100, Chicago, IL 60611-1676.

Of course, the Alzheimer's Association is not the only place that offers assistance to persons with dementia and their caregivers, and like any large national organization, it is not without its shortcomings. Many local groups also provide important and much-needed help, and it would be wise to seek support and information from as many sources as possible.

• • •

⟶ DEPRESSION ⟵

It probably does not come as a great surprise that a common lament among family members who care for relatives with dementia is similar to a statement heard at a support group meeting: "It's getting so I just can't believe this woman is my mother. It's so depressing." The problem, however, goes far beyond such colloquial expressions of discouragement to actual clinical depression, a much more serious *medical* condition than the normal and appropriate feelings of sadness we have in response to a difficult situation.

One study found that 55 percent of caregivers who shared a home with a demented person were clinically depressed—an amazingly high number. Other studies show that those caring for a person with dementia have three times as many stress symptoms as people of the same age who do not care for someone, use more drugs and alcohol (often taking the medicine prescribed to calm down the patient), and report lower satisfaction with life in general. As one 81-year-old who had been caring for his 79-year-old wife for a decade expressed it, "You never look happy, you never sound happy, your sleep is disturbed. She doesn't call me by name any more; she calls me 'mister.' I just try to make it through one day to the next."

With Alzheimer's disease, caregivers truly become patients, too. If you recognize yourself in the description above, please seek medical care. Depression is an illness that can be treated, and it is crucial for you to remember that you cannot provide the care you want to give your loved one if you are ill yourself.

In fact, a point that can hardly be stressed enough is that *caregivers have to care for themselves.* I have already talked about the importance of accepting help. Beyond that, one of the most crucial issues a caregiver must address is that of balancing the needs of your cognitively impaired loved one against your own (and sometimes against those of other family members as well). Many religious people feel they must be willing to sacrifice themselves for loved ones, even to the point of "laying down their lives" for them. I do not dispute the importance of such altruism, which lies at the heart of the Christian faith. As we have just seen, however, Alzheimer's disease makes patients of the entire family. If your primary concern is truly for the ill person, you simply must take care of yourself if you are to go on caring for him or her.

So I would like to "give you permission" here and now to take care of yourself, and I urge you to do so. You do not have to feel guilty if you get away for an afternoon or an evening (or even a whole day) every week; you are simply restoring yourself for the task at hand (remember that Jesus frequently withdrew "to a lonely place" for some revitalization when the demands of the crowds got to be too much for him). Look around for a good daycare or other type of respite program. Do not be afraid to ask family or friends to cover for you so you can have time away from your caregiving tasks. As one support group member said with a smile, "I had to go back to work four days a week to keep my husband in daycare five days, and I am happy to do it because I know I take better care of him when I'm there."

• • •

⤜∞⤏ **FEAR** ⤜∞⤏

Although fear plays a role in many of the topics just discussed, it is worthy of mention on its own because it is such a universal effect of caring for a demented relative. Fears prompted by diseases such as Alzheimer's are legion: fear the loved one will die; fear of one's own death first, leaving no one to care for the cognitively impaired individual; fear of financial problems or even ruin; fear of becoming unable to care for the person at home, thus necessitating institutionalization; fear of losing one's friends because of the ill person's strange behavior; and many others. These fears are real and often justified, and they need to be addressed in a practical way.

On a different level, however, do not overlook your religious faith as a rich source of material to help you face your fears. In the Hebrew Bible (Old Testament) you can find great strength and comfort in Psalms 23 and 27, as well as in many other less familiar Psalms. Indeed, this particular book of the Bible offers an especially valuable selection of verses and ideas that demonstrate quite clearly the timeless nature of the fears and other feelings that caregivers experience, as well as the fact that many people have found the strength to weather all kinds of threats and assaults in their vital faith in God (even though that faith is often tested and sometimes seems to be woefully inadequate). As a beginning, memorize and keep at hand for difficult moments the first verse of Psalm 46: "God is our refuge and strength, a very present help in time of trouble."

For Christians, of course, the New Testament also contains many familiar expressions of the comforting love and presence of Jesus Christ, such as John 14:1, 27 and Philippians 4:11-13, especially verse 13. Ask your clergyperson to suggest other texts that will help you and to discuss with you the meaning of any that are not clear.

Furthermore, do not fail to use one of the greatest resources believers have at their disposal in dealing with the terrible stress of caring for a person with dementia: the power of prayer. Tennyson was right when he said, "More things are wrought by prayer than this world dreams of." A serious prayer life can certainly bring you into closer relationship with the God who is the source of that "perfect love [that] casts out fear" (1 John 4:18). Although it has come to be associated with Alcoholics Anonymous, the so-called Serenity Prayer is a good source of strength and comfort to those who care for people with dementia, offering some very sound advice that may help you manage to maintain your sanity, even if it doesn't actually bring you serenity:

> *God grant me the serenity*
> *To accept the things I cannot change,*
> *The courage to change the things I can,*
> *And the wisdom to know the difference.*

Before closing this discussion, I want to mention the importance of continuing to include the ill person in religious observances, even after it appears that he or she is beyond comprehending what is going on. Many caregivers report that familiar rituals, prayers, Bible verses memorized decades earlier, and especially hymns prompt a strong response from people who otherwise seem completely inaccessible, and empirical research is beginning to support these personal observations. If this is the case, think how much comfort and reassurance people in early stages of Alzheimer's can receive from such sources! Indeed, entire worship services could be devised specifically for those with Alzheimer's disease and their families (see "Suggestions for Further Information" for a helpful resource). Even when the individual can no longer attend any kind of corporate worship, "that old, old story" can still be told and those old familiar hymns can still be played and sung.

POSITIVE ASPECTS OF CAREGIVING

I do not want to conclude this discussion of the impact of Alzheimer's disease on family caregivers without pointing out that even in the midst of the pain, stress, and turmoil, many caregivers discover some positive points. The nature of the illness itself, tragic as it is, allows a more positive light to be cast on the overall picture than is the case with unexpected death. With Alzheimer's disease, the lengthy period of deterioration that often seems so cruel also provides time to sort out, work through, and struggle for meaning and satisfaction in the caregiving task. In fact, caregivers have identified a number of positive aspects that can come from caring for a cognitively impaired loved one. Among the more commonly mentioned of these rewards of caregiving are the following:

- Pride in fulfilling one's obligations (e.g., living up to the marriage vow to love the spouse "in sickness and in health, for better and for worse, till death do us part," or returning to a beloved parent the care he or she provided the child when young)

- A heightened sense of self-worth coming from having done a difficult job well and from having provided a quality of care impossible to expect from anyone else

- The realization of a previously unknown ability to cope with an extremely rough situation, often primarily through the strength of one's own inner resources

- An enhanced closeness among family members who pitch in to help, and a greater appreciation for friends and others who offer support and assistance

- A renewed awareness of the wonder of the world as seen again through the eyes of the impaired loved one with an almost childlike appreciation of simple things

- And finally, but by no means last in importance, an increased spirituality and a closer relationship to God as the caregiver turns to his or her faith for support and meaning.

The struggle of caring for a loved one with Alzheimer's disease or other dementing illness is a long, hard one, and both the process and outcome are not what anyone would wish. But with a willingness to acknowledge your need for help—especially from the loving God who has promised to be with you always and who knows what it means to suffer for someone you love—the struggle can lead to new meaning and satisfaction in life, even amid the losses you feel so keenly.

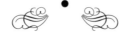

SUGGESTIONS FOR FURTHER INFORMATION

BOOKS:

Note: Since the first edition of this book was published in 1989, and even since the first revision in 1996, literature on Alzheimer's disease and particularly on caregiving issues has exploded. Perhaps the most helpful suggestion I can make here is that you go to the website of one of the large online booksellers (e.g., www.amazon.com or http://barnesandnoble.com) and search for "Alzheimer's." A wealth of resources will appear (a simple search at Amazon.com yielded 722 for me!). You can then look for the ones that strike you as most relevant for your needs. But I do want to mention just a few that you might start with.

Mitch Albom's book *Tuesdays with Morrie* (New York: Broadway Books, 2002) is not about Alzheimer's disease, but it is a remarkable memoir of "an old man, a young man, and life's greatest lesson" that will inspire and move anyone caring for and about another person at the end of life. See also Morrie Schwartz's *Letting Go: Morrie's Reflections on Living While Dying*

(New York: Dell, 1996) for more of Morrie's thoughtful words that can help the caregiver—and the person with early-stage Alzheimer's—face up to and respond positively to the inevitable outcome of the illness.

Virginia Bell's and David Troxel's book, *The Best Friends Approach to Alzheimer's Care* (Baltimore: Health Professions Press, 1996), is a creative and caring way to interact with people with dementia, including practical ways to handle common behavior problems.

The Loss of Self: A Family Resource for the Care of Alzheimer's Disease and Related Disorders (New York: W.W. Norton, revised and updated, 2002) by Donna Cohen and Carl Eisdorfer is an excellent "self-help" manual for family caregivers by two of the acknowledged authorities in the field. Likewise, their *Caring for Your Aging Parents: A Planning and Action Guide* (New York: J. P. Tarcher, 1995) is another helpful resource.

Wilfrid Gordon McDonald Partridge (La Jolla: Kane/Miller, 1995) by Mem Fox and Julie Vivas is a touching story about a little boy who lives next to a retirement home and sets out to find the memory of one of the elderly residents when she loses it. It is a wonderful book to introduce children to the world of Alzheimer's (and not a bad way to do so for adults).

Donna Guthrie's *Grandpa Doesn't Know It's Me* (New York: Human Sciences Press, 1986) is, sadly, out of print, but if you can find it in a used book store, it is another good resource to help young children understand dementia.

Lisa Gwyther's *You Are One of Us: Successful Clergy/Church Connections to Alzheimer's Families* (Duke Family Support Program, Box 3600 DUMC, Durham, N.C. 27710, 919-660-7510, 1995) is a valuable resource for clergy who want to help, and for caregivers who want to educate clergy and congregations in ways they *can* help!

Counting on Kindness: The Dilemmas of Dependency by Wendy Lustbader (New York: Free Press, 1994) is a heartening look at the difficult problem of what becoming dependent means for someone struggling with the loss of independence and for those who care about him or her.

Nancy Mace and Peter Rabins have updated for a second time *The 36-Hour Day: A Family Guide to Caring for Persons with Alzheimer's Disease, Related Dementing Illnesses, and Memory Loss in Later Life* (New York: Warner Books, 3rd edition, 2001), and it remains one of the best self-help books available, highly commended and widely used.

God Never Forgets: Faith, Hope, and Alzheimer's Disease (Louisville: Westminster John Knox Press, 1997), edited by Donald K. McKim, is a more scholarly, theological book for those who want to see how three contemporary religious scholars—professors of social work, biblical studies, and ethics—have used the resources of their specialties to try to understand the topics indicated in the subtitle.

Cecil Murphey's *My Parents, My Children: Spiritual Help for Caregivers* (Louisville: Westminster John Knox Press, 2000) is a useful book for connecting caregivers—especially those in the

"Sandwich Generation" who care simultaneously for elderly parents and children— with the greatest Source of help available to them.

James L. and Hilde L. Nelson's *Alzheimer's: Answers to Hard Questions for Families* (New York: Doubleday, 1996) is a step-by-step guide to caring for a loved one with Alzheimer's, presented through hypothetical scenes portraying some of the common situations caregivers face. Be forewarned, though, that some readers find the authors' approach overly judgmental and neglectful of some of the long-term impacts on family caregivers.

Worship Services for People with Alzheimer's Disease: A Handbook, edited by Elizabeth Pohlman and Gloria Bloom (Eddy Alzheimer's Disease Assistance Center, 2220 Burdett Avenue, Troy, New York 12180), is a useful guide for individuals and religious institutions who want to hold worship experiences for cognitively impaired persons.

Marty Richards' *Caregiving: Church and Family Together* (Louisville: Geneva Press, 1999) contains a more detailed look at some of this issues addressed in this book, with helpful advice for caregivers and congregations in a format that can be used as a study guide for group discussion.

Caring for Those with Alzheimer's: A Pastoral Approach by Joan D. Roberts (Staten Island, New York: Alba House, 2000) contains practical tips for caregivers and good information for clergy and counselors.

Now out of print, Stephen Sapp's *Full of Years: Aging and the Elderly in the Bible and Today* (Nashville: Abingdon Press, 1987) is a useful overview of aging and our responsibilities toward the elderly from a biblical perspective.

Catch a Falling Star: Living with Alzheimer's by Betty Baker Spohr with Jean Valens Bullard (Seattle: Storm Peak Press, 1995) is a very personal narrative of a caregiver's journey presented in straightforward, engaging, and sometimes humorous terms, celebrating the human spirit and its qualities that make something as insidious as Alzheimer's manageable. A page of "Points to Remember" at the end of each chapter offers helpful tips that enable caregivers to be spared many problems as the disease progresses that the author learned to handle through often painful experience.

• • •

ORGANIZATIONS:

In addition to the Alzheimer's Association mentioned in the text, several other excellent sources of useful information for caregivers and others are easily accessible:

Alzheimer's Disease Education and Referral Center (part of the National Institute on Aging of the National Institutes of Health), PO Box 8250, Silver Spring, MD 20907-8250 (800-438-4380 or www.alzheimers.org), provides a wealth of information on all aspects of Alzheimer's, including referrals for services and materials, research updates, a comprehensive bibliographic database, the clinical trials database mentioned earlier, and an e-mail address (adear@alzheimers.org) where information specialists will answer your questions about Alzheimer's disease.

Children of Aging Parents, 1609 Woodbourne Road, Suite 302A, Levittown, PA 19057-1511 (800-227-7294 or www.caps4caregivers.org), is a nonprofit group that provides information and materials for adult children caring for their older parents. Caregivers of people with Alzheimer's disease also may find this information helpful.

Eldercare Locator (800-677-1116 or www.eldercare.gov) is a nationwide referral service funded by the federal Administration on Aging (AoA) that assists elders and their caregivers in finding local support and resources. AoA also offers a helpful resource for caregivers called *Because We Care: A Guide for People Who Care* (available at www.aoa.gov/wecare/default.htm). AoA's Alzheimer's Disease Resource Room (www.aoa.gov/alz/index.asp) contains information for families, caregivers, professionals, and providers about Alzheimer's disease, caregiving, working with and providing services to people with Alzheimer's, and sources of help.

The National Council on the Aging (NCOA) offer a wonderful, easy-to-use online service called *BenefitsCheckUp* (www.benefitscheckup.org) that can help you determine what services the person you are caring for (or you yourself) might be entitled to. This free, confidential tool is designed specifically for elders and caregivers and searches more than 1,000 federal and state programs to find those for which you may be eligible. This is a resource that you simply must take advantage of!

NOTES

[1] - The medical profession's name for this illness is evolving to "Alzheimer disease," as occurred with the transition from Down's syndrome to Down syndrome. I have chosen to retain the more familiar form in this book.

[2] - Median age is the age at which half the population being examined is older and half is younger. It is a more accurate statistical measure of age composition than average age.

[3] - *Brain Failure: An Introduction to Current Concepts of Senility* (New York: Free Press, 1981).

[4] - Donna Cohen and Carl Eisdorfer, *The Loss of Self: A Family Resource for the Care of Alzheimer's Disease and Related Disorders* (New York: W.W. Norton, 1986), p. 146.

[5] - The question of the cause(s) of Alzheimer's disease is an extremely complex one and far beyond the scope of this book. If you are interested in knowing more, you can easily find a

great deal of information on the topic, beginning with the websites listed under "Suggestions for Further Information." For a comprehensible overview of recent research into Alzheimer's disease, see the *Time* article mentioned earlier in the text (July 17, 2000), as well as another article in the January 31, 2000, issue.

[6] - One study showed a 93 percent accuracy rate when diagnoses of experienced neurologists were compared to autopsy findings.

[7] - In 2001, for example, the Association of the British Pharmaceutical Industry published a booklet (*Targeting Alzheimer's*) that describes over 30 treatment and preventive possibilities being developed at various drug companies or academic medical centers around the world.

[8] - The National Institute on Aging (NIA) and the Food and Drug Administration (FDA) maintain the Alzheimer's Disease Clinical Trials Database, which lists clinical trials sponsored by the government and by private pharmaceutical companies. You can learn about these studies by contacting the NIA's Alzheimer's Disease Education and Referral Center (ADEAR) at 800-438-4380 or by visiting ADEAR's Alzheimer's Disease Clinical Trials Database at www.alzheimers.org/trials.index.html. You may want to check regularly to learn what new drug studies have been added to the database.

[9] - See Stephen Sapp, *Full of Years: Aging and the Elderly in the*

Bible and Today (Nashville: Abingdon Press, 1987), pp. 81-88, 179-192, for a discussion of the meaning and contemporary application of this crucial commandment.

[10] - This experience reminds me of the story of the two physicians riding together to a medical society meeting. One said, "I bet we have roast beef, baked potatoes with butter and sour cream, and cheesecake for dessert. With all we know about fat, cholesterol, and their link to stroke and heart disease, you'd think a medical association would choose banquet menus more carefully." His friend agreed, and their conversation turned to other matters, including the likely increase in dementing illnesses that will accompany the aging of the population of the United States in the coming decades. They began to share experiences they had had with Alzheimer's patients and their families, and by the time they got to the banquet both of them asked for seconds on the prime rib, butter, and cheesecake!

[11] - See Sapp, Full of Years, chapter 4, for further development of this idea.

[12] - This is an area that is especially difficult for many caregivers, and one that is fraught with emotion and misconceptions, not least on the part of healthcare professionals. This is not the place for a detailed discussion of the matter, but I urge you to give it serious thought and to discuss it frankly with family members and your loved one's physician before it becomes an issue.

[13] - For this distinction, I am indebted to Harley Swiggum,

author of the Bethel Series Adult Bible Study Program of the Adult Christian Education Foundation, Madison, Wisconsin. I have altered Mr. Swiggum's original usage somewhat.

[14] - *Letting Go: Morrie's Reflections on Living While Dying* (New York: Dell, 1996), pp. 106-107.

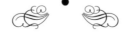

Is It Alzheimer's? Ten Warning Signs

This checklist was developed by the Alzheimer's Association to help family members and others know what warning signs to look for if you are concerned about the behavior of a loved one or friend. If several are present, the person should see a physician for a complete examination.

1. **Recent memory loss that affects job performance.** Occasional forgetting is normal. People with Alzheimer's may forget they asked the same question, not remember the answer, or that they asked the question.
2. **Difficulty performing familiar tasks.** Busy people forget sometimes. People with Alzheimer's could prepare a meal, forget to serve it, and even forget that they made it.
3. **Problems with language.** They may forget simple words or substitute inappropriate words, making their sentences incomprehensible.
4. **Disorientation to time and place.** People with Alzheimer's disease can get lost on their own street, not knowing where they are, how they got there, or how to get home.
5. **Poor or decreased judgment.** Example: Forgetting a child

under his or her care and leaving the house to visit a neighbor.

6. **Problems with abstract thinking.** Someone with Alzheimer's could forget what the numbers in a checkbook are and what needs to be done with them.

7. **Misplacing things.** We all misplace things. The person with Alzheimer's may put things in inappropriate places—an iron in the freezer, a watch in the sugar bowl—and not be able to retrieve them.

8. **Changes in mood or behavior.** Someone with Alzheimer's can exhibit rapid mood swings for no apparent reason, e.g., from calm, to tears, to anger, and back to calm in a few minutes.

9. **Changes in personality.** A person with Alzheimer's disease can change drastically, becoming extremely irritable, suspicious, or fearful.

10. **Loss of initiative.** The person with Alzheimer's may become very passive and require cues and prompting to get involved in activities.

These warning signs may apply to dementias other than Alzheimer's disease. People concerned about these warning signs should see a physician familiar with dementias.

Reprinted by permission of the Alzheimer's Association.

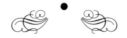

Ten Warning Signs of Caregiver Stress

This helpful list of signs to watch out for in caregivers of people with dementia was compiled by the Alzheimer's Association. If you are a caregiver and recognize yourself below, or if you know a caregiver who is showing these signs, please seek assistance. Remember: Caregivers cannot provide care if they don't take care of themselves!

1. **Denial**—about the disease and its effects on the person who's been diagnosed. *I know mom's going to get better.*
2. **Anger**—at the person with Alzheimer's or others: that no effective treatments or cures currently exist, and that people don't understand what's going on. *If he asks me that question one more time I'll scream!*
3. **Social withdrawal**—from friends and activities that once brought pleasure. *I don't care about getting together with the neighbors anymore.*
4. **Anxiety**—about facing another day and what the future holds. *What happens when he needs more care than I can provide?*
5. **Depression**—begins to break your spirit and affects your ability to cope. *I don't care anymore.*
6. **Exhaustion**—makes it nearly impossible to complete neces-

sary daily tasks. *I'm too tired for this.*

7. **Sleeplessness**—caused by a never-ending list of concerns. *What if she wanders out of the house or falls and hurts herself?*

8. **Irritability**—leads to moodiness and triggers negative responses and reactions. *Leave me alone!*

9. **Lack of concentration**—makes it difficult to perform familiar tasks. *I was so busy, I forgot we had an appointment.*

10. **Health problems**—begin to take their toll, both mentally and physically. *I can't remember the last time I felt good.*

Reprinted by permission of the Alzheimer's Association.

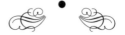

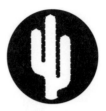

DESERT MINISTRIES INCORPORATED

Desert Ministries is a non-profit corporation devoted to the development of helpful materials for use by those in special need. It provides books and booklets for clergy and for laity on a variety of subjects. Information on other publications will be sent upon request. A sample packet will be sent without charge if you ask.

Recent publications include: *When You Lose Someone You Love, How to Help an Alcoholic, Christ Will See You Through, God's Promises and My Needs, You Now Have Custody of You, When Alzheimer's Strikes, When a Child Dies,* and more.

Desert Ministries, Inc.
P.O. Box 788
Palm Beach, FL 33480

www.desmin.org